LET'S BUILD CHAMPIONS

Complete Strength & Conditioning Guide for Combat Sports

BY

LARRY WADE

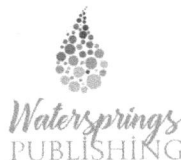

Watersprings
PUBLISHING

Let's Build Champions by Larry Wade
Published by Watersprings Publishing,
P.O. Box 1284 Olive Branch, MS 38654
www.waterspringspublishing.com

Contact the publisher for bulk orders and permission requests.

Printed in the United States of America.

ISBN-13: 978-1-964972-12-1

LET'S BUILD CHAMPIONS

PREFACE

Boxing is a sport that pushes the human body and mind to its limits. It is a test of endurance, strength, speed, and resilience. Throughout history, the sport has evolved from unstructured bare-knuckle brawls to a sophisticated discipline that requires not only technical prowess but also elite physical conditioning.

Yet, for far too long, strength and conditioning were overlooked in boxing. Fighters relied solely on skills and heart to carry them through battles, often neglecting the physical preparation that could give them a competitive edge. In recent decades, however, this has changed. The modern fighter is expected to be a complete athlete, and that means integrating strength, power, and endurance into their training regimens.

As a coach, my job is to build champions. My journey into strength and conditioning didn't begin in the boxing gym—it started on the track, where speed, power, and endurance are the foundation of success. My experience as a world-class track and field athlete, competing at the highest levels, taught me how to push the body to its limits and beyond. That experience has shaped my approach to training fighters, blending explosive athleticism with combat-specific conditioning to create elite-level boxers.

In this book, I will share the knowledge and methodologies I've developed over the years, working with some of the best fighters in the world. This is not just a book about lifting weights or running sprints; this is about understanding the science behind peak performance in boxing. Whether you're a coach, a fighter, or simply a fan of the sport, my goal is to provide you with the tools and insights needed to train smarter, perform better, and achieve success in the ring.

Welcome to the journey.

Coach Larry Wade
"I Build Champions"

INTRODUCTION

The Evolution of Strength and Conditioning in Boxing

Boxing's Early Days: Natural Ability Over Training

In the early years of boxing, dating back to the 17th century in Britain, there was little emphasis on structured training. Fighters relied on their raw physicality, toughness, and instincts to survive brutal contests. With no gloves, few rules, and no governing bodies to regulate training, most boxers simply fought with what they had.

The first recorded boxing match took place on January 6, 1681, when Christopher Monck, 2nd Duke of Albemarle, arranged a fight between his butler and his butcher. Matches like these were not about athletic training—they were brutal brawls, often fought to the death. It wasn't until the mid-1800s that boxing began to take a more organized form. The Marquess of Queensberry Rules, established in 1867, brought order to the sport by introducing gloves, timed rounds, and weight classes. While these changes helped shape modern boxing, physical conditioning remained a secondary concern.

The Rise of Strength & Conditioning in Boxing

For much of the 20th century, boxing training was rooted in tradition. Fighters relied on roadwork, shadowboxing, bag work, and sparring. Strength training was often discouraged, with the belief that lifting weights would slow a fighter down or make them too bulky.

It wasn't until the late 1960s that strength and conditioning began to gain recognition in combat sports. Pioneers like Alvin Roy and Mackie Shilstone introduced strength training principles that helped boxers develop explosive power, endurance, and resilience. By the late 20th century, the role of strength and conditioning coaches became indispensable for elite fighters.

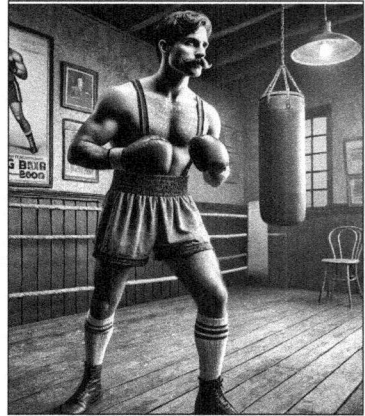

Today, boxing training is more advanced than ever. Fighters no longer rely solely on roadwork and bag drills; they incorporate strength training, plyometrics, agility drills, sports science, and data-driven training programs to optimize their performance. The modern fighter is expected to be an elite athlete, finely tuned to handle the demands of championship-level competition.

Why I Wrote This Book

My transition into boxing was unexpected but inevitable. Coming from an elite track and field background, I understood how to maximize an athlete's speed, power, and endurance. When I was introduced to the sport of boxing, I saw a gap—a need for structured, science-based strength and conditioning programs tailored specifically for fighters.

One experience, in particular, made me realize just how crucial proper training is. In 2019, at the University of Nevada, Las Vegas (UNLV) track, I witnessed a young fighter being pushed beyond safe limits in extreme heat.

His coach had him running 10 sets of 400-meter sprints with only a minute of rest between each—a dangerous workout given the 110-115°F temperatures. By the fourth sprint, the fighter collapsed from exhaustion. His heart rate was dangerously high, 220 beats per minute, far exceeding safe thresholds.

This wasn't training—it was recklessness. It was then that I realized how many fighters were being put through ineffective, outdated, and sometimes dangerous training methods by coaches who lacked proper knowledge of sports science.

This book is my way of bridging the gap between traditional boxing training and modern strength and conditioning science. Fighters need to be trained efficiently, safely, and with purpose. My goal is to ensure that no athlete is ever put in a situation where their health is compromised due to ignorance, misinformation, or poor coaching.

Who is This Book For?

This book is for fighters, coaches, trainers, and anyone looking to understand the science behind boxing performance. Whether you're a young prospect, a seasoned veteran, or a coach wanting to improve your athletes' performance, you will find valuable insights here.

- If you are a fighter, this book will teach you how to train smarter, get stronger, and improve your conditioning without sacrificing speed or mobility.

- If you are a coach, this book will help you develop structured, effective training plans that maximize your fighter's potential.

- If you are a fan of the sport, this book will give you an inside look at the physical preparation that separates champions from contenders.

What Will You Learn?

In the pages ahead, we'll cover everything from strength training and energy system development to recovery and injury prevention. You'll learn about:

- The three body types (Ectomorph, Mesomorph, Endomorph) and how they affect training.

- How the body's energy systems work and why they matter in boxing.

- The difference between aerobic, anaerobic, and explosive power training.

- How to structure a fighter's training camp (Pre-Camp, Camp, and Post-Camp).

- The dangers of improper weight-cutting and how to do it safely.

- How heart rate monitoring can optimize training and recovery.

- Lessons from coaching World Champions like Shawn Porter, Badou Jack, and Caleb Plant.

Boxing is evolving, and so must its training methods. This book is designed to equip you with the knowledge, tools, and strategies needed to train at the highest level. Whether your goal is to win a world title, improve your fitness, or train fighters effectively, the information contained within these pages will serve as your blueprint. So, are you ready to take your training to the next level? Let's begin.

A well-structured strength and conditioning program enhances every aspect of a boxer's performance.

CHAPTER 1
The Role of Strength & Conditioning in Boxing

Why Strength & Conditioning is Essential for Fighters

For years, the world of boxing resisted change when it came to physical preparation. Traditional training methods—roadwork, bag drills, and sparring—were seen as the only necessary tools to build a fighter. Strength training was often dismissed as something that would slow a boxer down or make them stiff. But as boxing evolved and competition became fiercer, it became clear that fighters needed more than just technical skills and grit—they needed to be complete athletes.

The Old-School Mentality

The boxing greats of the past—fighters like Muhammad Ali, Joe Frazier, and Sugar Ray Leonard—built their endurance through countless miles of roadwork, their speed through endless rounds of mitt work, and their strength through calisthenics and sparring. There was little emphasis on strength and conditioning beyond bodyweight exercises and general fitness.

The idea of lifting weights or using structured strength programs was frowned upon. Many trainers believed that lifting would make a boxer slow, bulky, and inflexible. Fighters relied on their natural abilities, their toughness, and their relentless training in the ring. While this approach worked in the past, modern boxing has shown that a scientifically backed, structured approach to strength and conditioning gives fighters a clear advantage.

The Shift to Modern Training

By the late 20th century, sports science had revolutionized training across all sports, including boxing. Fighters and coaches began to realize that strength, speed, endurance, and power could be trained systematically to enhance performance. The top fighters in the world today—whether it's Shawn Porter, Badou Jack, or Caleb Plant—incorporate strength training, sprint work, plyometrics, and advanced recovery methods into their camps.

Modern strength and conditioning for boxing isn't about bulking up or trying to lift the heaviest weights— it's about training specifically for boxing. That means:

- **Explosive power** to generate knockout punches.
- **Speed and agility** to move fluidly around the ring.
- **Endurance** to sustain high work rates for 12 rounds.

- **Core strength and stability** to take punches and maintain balance.

- **Injury prevention** to extend careers and keep fighters in peak condition.

How Strength & Conditioning Transforms a Boxer

A well-structured strength and conditioning program enhances every aspect of a boxer's performance. Here's how:

1. Increased Punching Power

One of the biggest misconceptions is that punching power is purely genetic. While some fighters are naturally heavy-handed, power can be developed through explosive strength training. Exercises like medicine ball slams, plyometric push-ups, kettlebell swings, and Olympic lifts train the fast-twitch muscle fibers that generate knockout power.

2. Improved Endurance and Recovery

Boxing is one of the most physically demanding sports, requiring both aerobic (long-duration) and anaerobic (short-burst) conditioning. A proper strength and conditioning program ensures that a fighter:

- Maintains high energy levels in later rounds.

- Recovers quickly between explosive

movements.

- Does not cause fatigue from throwing punches or absorbing blows.

Interval training, sprint work, and heart rate-based conditioning help fighters develop fight-specific endurance.

3. Faster Footwork and Agility

Footwork is the foundation of boxing. Fighters must be able to move quickly, cut angles, evade punches, and explode into offensive or defensive movements. A well-trained fighter moves efficiently and effortlessly across the ring. Agility drills, ladder work, and resistance band training enhance a fighter's movement patterns, making them faster and more elusive.

4. Greater Injury Resistance

Boxing is brutal on the body. Without proper strength training, fighters are more prone to injuries like:

- Hand fractures from poor punch mechanics.
- Shoulder injuries from repetitive strain.
- Lower back and core weakness affecting balance.
- Knee and ankle issues from poor foot positioning.

A strength and conditioning program strengthens

muscles, ligaments, and joints, helping fighters withstand the rigors of the sport and stay healthier longer.

5. Improved Weight Management and Body Composition

Boxing is a weight-class sport, meaning fighters must control their body composition carefully. Strength and conditioning, combined with proper nutrition, helps:

- Increase lean muscle mass without excessive bulk.

- Reduce unnecessary body fat.

- Optimize hydration and performance leading up to weigh-ins.

Fighters who cut weight incorrectly often lose strength and endurance, which is why a structured training plan ensures they stay strong and conditioned while making weight safely.

Breaking the Myth: "Strength Training Will Make You Slow"

One of the biggest misconceptions in boxing is that lifting weights makes you slow. This myth has been debunked countless times in modern sports science. When done correctly, strength training actually makes fighters:

- Faster

- More explosive

- More efficient with their movements

Training methods like plyometrics, resistance sprinting, and Olympic weightlifting are designed to enhance speed, not hinder it. The key is focusing on:

- Explosive, fast lifts (not slow, heavy bodybuilding movements).

- Dynamic, full-body movements (not isolated muscle training).

- Sport-specific drills that transfer directly to boxing performance.

Case Study: The Transformation of Shawn Porter

Shawn Porter is a prime example of how strength and conditioning can change a fighter's career. Shawn was a talented boxer with relentless pressure with explosiveness and endurance.

By implementing track-based sprint training, explosive weightlifting, and strategic conditioning drills, Kenny Porter (Head Trainer) and I were able to transform his:

- Cardiovascular endurance

- Power output

- Speed and agility

The Result

Shawn Porter became a two time World Champion and one of the best fighters in the world. Having the opportunity to fight other great fighters such as Keith Thurman, Danny Garcia, Errol Spence, and Terrence Crawford. His ability to maintain high-pressure fighting for 12 rounds was largely due to his elite conditioning.

What Fighters and Coaches Need to Understand

Strength and conditioning should NEVER replace traditional boxing training—but it should be an integral part of every fighter's routine. The best fighters in the world combine their technical skill with world-class

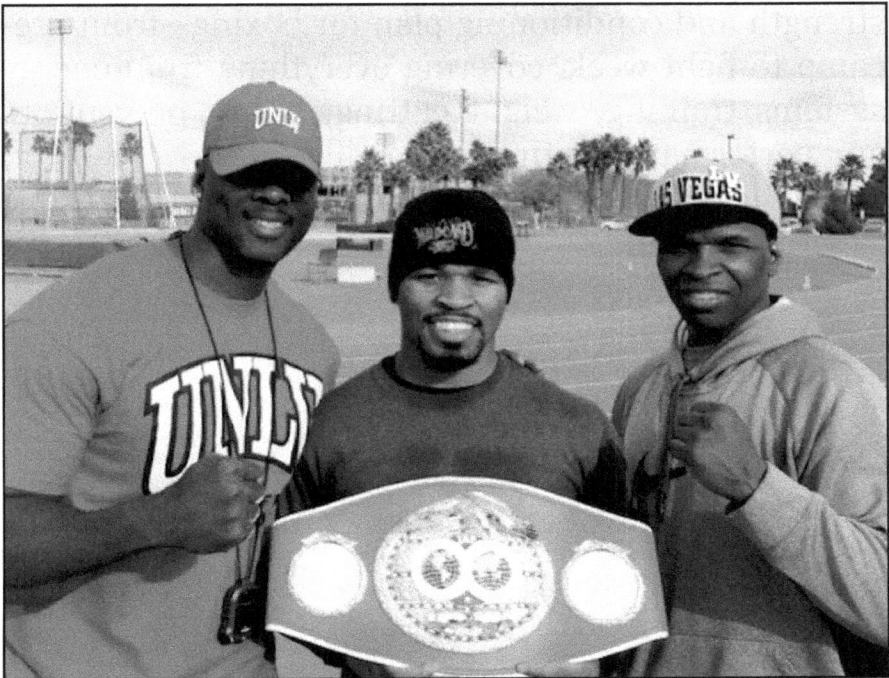

conditioning to ensure they are as prepared as possible on fight night.

A well-rounded program will:

1. **Optimize strength and power** for punching and movement.

2. **Improve speed and agility** to outmaneuver opponents.

3. **Enhance endurance** to sustain high-energy output for 12 rounds.

4. **Prevent injuries** and prolong careers.

5. **Ensure fighters are making weight safely and effectively.**

This book will break down how to develop a complete strength and conditioning plan for boxing—from pre-camp to fight week, covering everything from energy systems training, weight cutting, injury prevention, and performance optimization.

CHAPTER 2

The Three Body Types & Their Impact on Training

Boxers come in all shapes and sizes, from the long and lean Tommy Hearns to the stocky and powerful Mike Tyson. While skills and training play a massive role in a fighter's success, genetics also influence how a boxer develops physically. A fighter's body type—whether they are naturally lean, muscular, or stocky—affects their strength, endurance, metabolism, and overall conditioning approach.

In this chapter, we'll break down the three primary body types in boxing:

1. **Ectomorphs** – Lean and long

2. **Mesomorphs** – Athletic and muscular

3. **Endomorphs** – Heavy, Stocky, and powerful

Understanding body types allows fighters and coaches to tailor strength, conditioning, and nutrition plans for optimal performance.

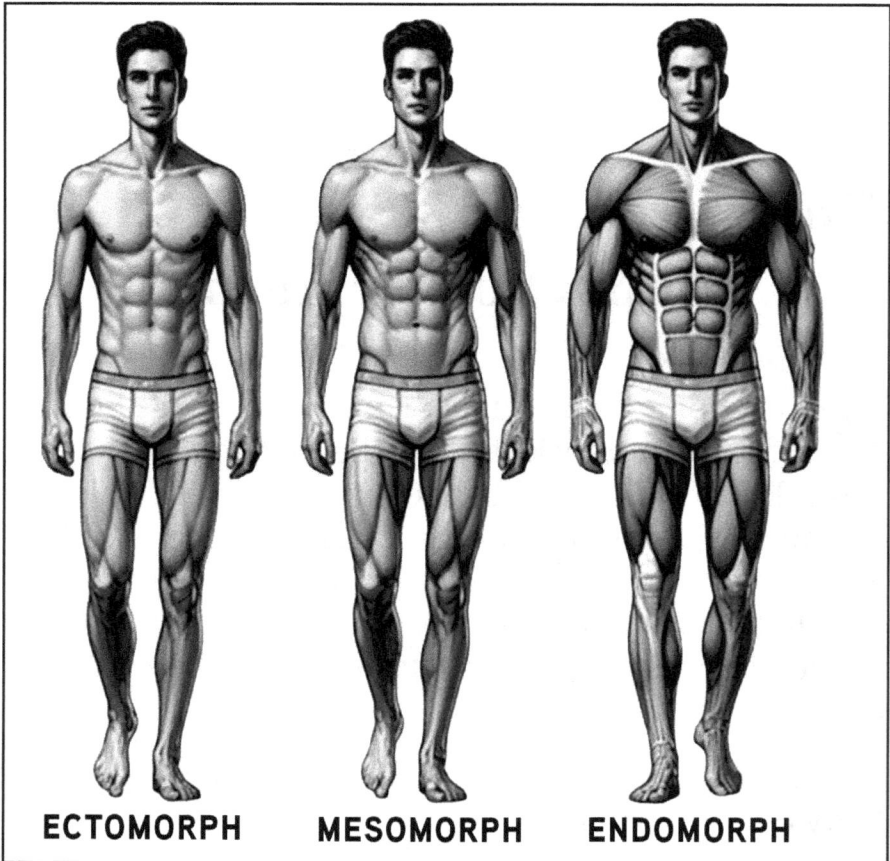

ECTOMORPH   MESOMORPH   ENDOMORPH

Why Body Type Matters in Boxing

Every fighter has a unique physique that influences how they move, how much energy they expend, and how they gain or lose weight. Here's why body type is important:

- **Different energy needs** – Some fighters burn calories faster than others.

- **Training adaptations** – Certain fighters build strength easier, while others struggle with endurance.

- **Weight management** – Cutting or gaining weight can be more difficult for some body types.

- **Fighting style influence** – A naturally explosive fighter will have different conditioning needs than a volume puncher.

Coaches who fail to consider body type often apply one-size-fits-all training that doesn't work for every athlete. This chapter will show you how to train smarter based on a fighter's body composition.

1. The Ectomorph Body Type: The Natural Endurance Fighter

Characteristics:

- Long limbs, lean frame

- Fast metabolism (struggles to gain weight)

- Naturally lower muscle mass

- High endurance but lower strength

- Typically found in lighter weight classes

Ectomorphs are naturally lean and built for endurance. Fighters in this category have long arms and legs, giving them a reach advantage, but they often lack raw power and muscle density. They excel in high-volume, high-work rate fighting—think fighters like Paul Williams or Tommy Hearns, who overwhelmed opponents with activity rather than knockout power.

Training for Ectomorphs

Strength & Power Focus

Because ectomorphs struggle with strength and muscle mass, they need progressive strength training while avoiding excessive endurance work.

- Heavy weightlifting (low reps, high weight)

- Explosive exercises (power cleans, kettle bell swings, plyometrics)

- Lower endurance volume (to avoid overtraining their natural strength)

- Too much cardio – Since they already have a strong aerobic system, excess roadwork can burn muscle mass.

- Low-weight, high-rep lifting – Won't develop the necessary power for knockout punches.

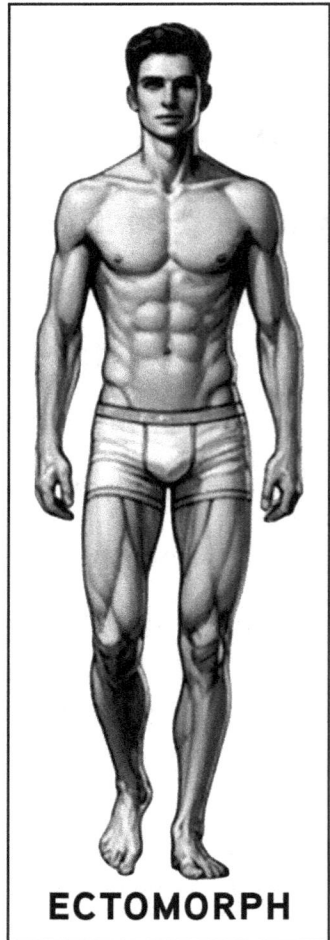

ECTOMORPH

Conditioning Focus

Ectomorphs should prioritize speed and power development rather than excessive endurance work.

- Sprint training (200m & 400m sprints)
- Short, intense conditioning rounds (battle ropes, sled pushes)
- Focus on explosive power instead of long-distance running

Nutrition Strategy

Ectomorphs burn calories very quickly. If they don't eat enough, they'll struggle to maintain muscle.

- High-calorie intake (quality carbs & protein)
- Frequent meals to avoid muscle loss
- Proper hydration to prevent energy dips

Famous Ectomorph Fighters:

- Tommy Hearns (Tall, lean frame with elite endurance)
- Paul Williams (High work rate, long reach)
- Michael Spinks (Naturally thin, but developed knockout power through strength training)

2. The Mesomorph Body Type: The Ideal Boxer's Physique

Characteristics:

- Naturally muscular and well-balanced

- Gains muscle and strength easily

- Moderate metabolism (can gain or lose weight with ease)

- Explosive and powerful, yet retains endurance

- Found in all weight classes

- Mesomorphs are genetically gifted athletes.

- They are strong, powerful, and agile, making them the perfect body type for boxing.

- Fighters like Shawn Porter and Mike Tyson exemplify mesomorph physiques— muscular, explosive, and capable of sustained pressure fighting.

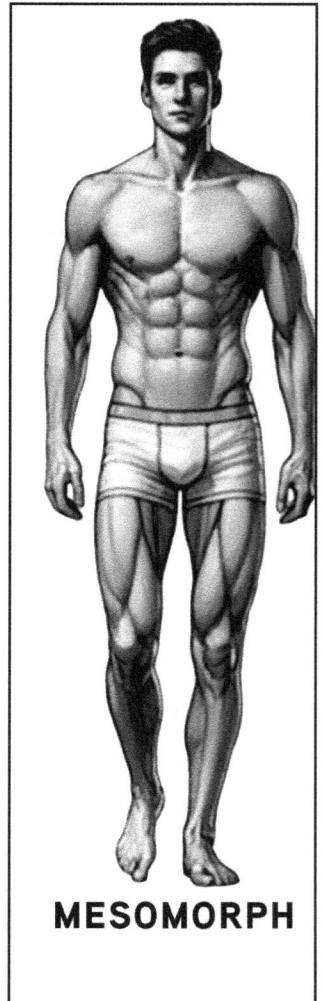

MESOMORPH

Training for Mesomorphs

Strength & Power Focus

Mesomorphs naturally build muscle, but they must balance strength training with maintaining flexibility and endurance.

- Moderate weightlifting (not too heavy, not too light)

- Explosive strength training (medicine ball throws, sprint resistance training)

- Bodyweight and agility training (to avoid becoming stiff)

- Excessive heavy lifting – Can reduce flexibility and slow reaction time.

- Ignoring mobility – If they don't stretch and work on agility, they can become stiff.

Conditioning Focus

Mesomorphs need a mix of endurance and explosive training.

- Interval training (high-intensity bursts with rest periods)

- Shadowboxing with resistance bands (to maintain speed and endurance)

- Footwork drills to ensure mobility isn't compromised by muscle gain

Nutrition Strategy

Mesomorphs can gain or lose weight easily. Their focus should be on lean muscle maintenance.

- Balanced diet (moderate carbs, high protein, healthy fats)
- Pre-fight weight adjustments based on body composition needs
- Adequate hydration for muscle recovery

Famous Mesomorph Fighters:

- Shawn Porter (Relentless pressure fighter with a strong build)
- Gervonta Davis (Explosive, powerful, yet mobile)
- Canelo Álvarez (Muscular but maintains endurance)

3. The Endomorph Body Type: The Natural Heavyweight

Characteristics:

- Stocky, solid frame with broad shoulders
- Slower metabolism (gains weight easily)
- Naturally strong but struggles with endurance
- Powerful puncher, high durability
- Found mostly in heavyweight and cruiserweight divisions

Endomorphs are built for power and durability. Fighters like Tyson Fury and Andy Ruiz Jr. carry extra weight but still perform at an elite level. Their natural strength and toughness make them formidable opponents, even if they don't appear as lean as other fighters.

Training for Endomorphs

Strength & Power Focus

Endomorphs are naturally strong but must train for explosive speed to avoid being too slow.

- Speed-focused weight training (explosive squats, trap bar deadlifts)

- Plyometrics (jump squats, sprint drills)

- Functional strength exercises (sled pushes, tire flips)

- Heavy, slow lifting without speed work – Can make them sluggish.

- Over-reliance on strength without agility drills – Leads to poor mobility in fights.

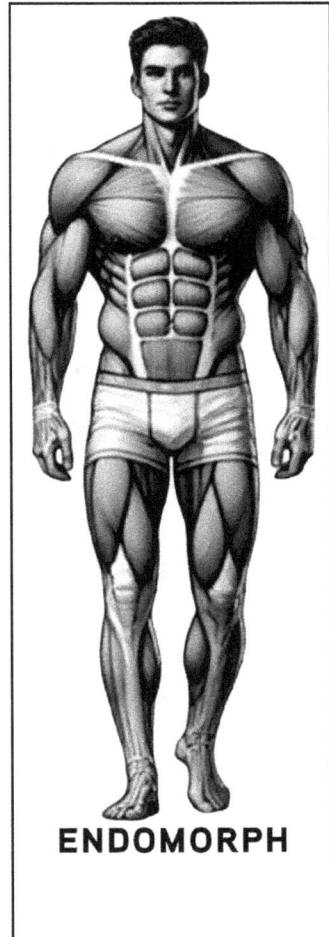

ENDOMORPH

Conditioning Focus

Endomorphs need to prioritize stamina training to avoid gassing out.

- High-intensity interval training (short bursts, minimal rest)

- Lighter, fast-paced footwork drills

- Extended endurance sessions (longer rounds to improve stamina)

Nutrition Strategy

Endomorphs must carefully monitor weight while ensuring energy levels remain high.

- Controlled carbohydrate intake (to prevent excess fat gain)

- High-protein, low-sugar diet

- Hydration focus (to avoid sluggishness in fights)

Famous Endomorph Fighters:

- Tyson Fury (Large frame, yet mobile and skilled)

- Andy Ruiz Jr. (Explosive hand speed despite heavier weight)

- Joe Frazier (Stocky, powerful inside fighter)

Conclusion: Using Body Type to Maximize Performance

By understanding a fighter's body type, coaches and athletes can:

- Optimize training for strength, power, and endurance

- Structure nutrition plans for better weight management

- Develop personalized conditioning routines for maximum efficiency

Coaches who fail to consider body type often apply one-size-fits-all training that doesn't work for every athlete.

CHAPTER 3
Understanding Energy Systems in Boxing

Boxing is one of the most physically demanding sports in the world. A single round requires bursts of explosive power, sustained endurance, quick recovery between exchanges, and the ability to maintain focus and technical sharpness even under extreme fatigue.

To train effectively for boxing, fighters must understand how their body produces energy. The body doesn't just run on one energy system—it cycles through three primary energy systems that fuel different types of movement.

In this chapter, we'll break down:

1. The Aerobic Energy System (Long-duration endurance)

2. The Anaerobic Lactic Energy System (High-intensity bursts, short-duration)

3. The Anaerobic Alactic Energy System (Explosive, short bursts of energy)

By understanding these energy systems, fighters and coaches can design optimized training programs that develop endurance, speed, power, and recovery.

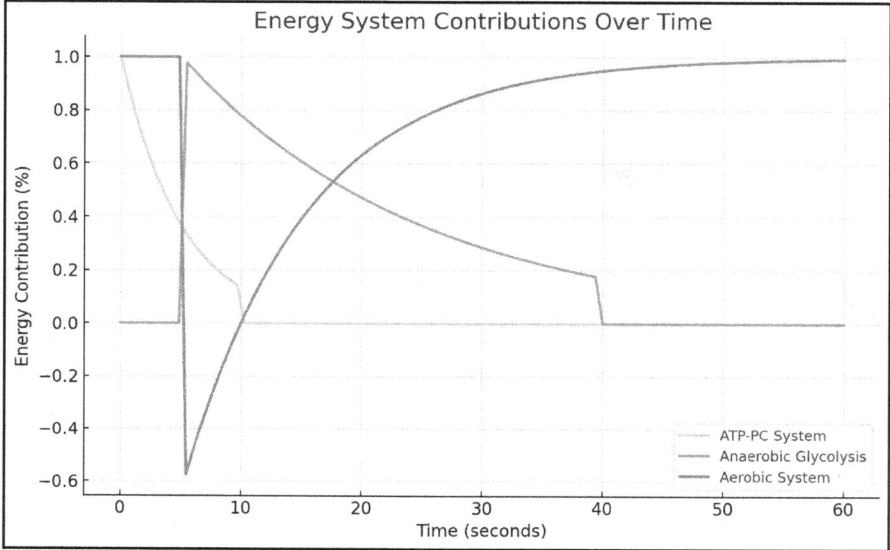

Energy System Contributions Over Time

Why Energy Systems Matter in Boxing

A boxing match is not a marathon, but it's also not a sprint. Each round is a blend of explosive power, sustained movement, and strategic pacing. Fighters who fail to train all three energy systems will find themselves gassing out, losing power, or struggling to recover during a fight.

The Three Phases of a Round:

Explosive Movements – Throwing a power punch, reacting to an opponent's shot, or slipping and countering. (Anaerobic Alactic System)

Sustained High-Intensity Exchanges – Trading punches in a combination, fighting inside the pocket, or engaging in a fast-paced round. (Anaerobic Lactic System)

Recovery & Movement – Circling the ring, light jabs, moving strategically, and catching breath between exchanges. (Aerobic System)

Each of these phases is powered by a different energy system. If one system is weak, a fighter's overall performance suffers.

1. The Aerobic Energy System (Long-Duration Endurance)

What it Does:

The *aerobic system* fuels sustained activity over long periods. This system is active whenever you're performing low-to-moderate-intensity work, such as jogging, moving around the ring, and light shadowboxing.

Why it's Important in Boxing:

- Supports overall endurance and allows a fighter to maintain energy throughout a 12-round fight.
- Improves recovery between rounds and between high-intensity exchanges.
- Prevents fatigue build-up by supplying oxygen to the muscles.

How to Train the Aerobic System:

- Long-Distance Running (Roadwork) – 3 to 6 miles at a steady pace.

- Shadowboxing Rounds – 4-6 rounds at moderate pace, focusing on breathing control.

- Jump Rope – 10-15 minutes at a steady rhythm to build cardiovascular endurance.

Common Mistakes:

- Too much slow, steady-state running without high-intensity work.

- Ignoring breathing efficiency—fighters must learn to control their breathing to maximize oxygen intake.

- Over-reliance on the aerobic system—boxing is not just about endurance, it also requires explosive energy.

When the Aerobic System Fails:

If a fighter lacks a strong aerobic system, they'll struggle to recover between rounds and between explosive movements. They may start strong but fade in the later rounds due to inefficient energy use.

2. The Anaerobic Lactic Energy System (High-Intensity, Short Duration)

What It Does:

The anaerobic lactic system provides energy for high-intensity movements lasting between 30 seconds to two minutes. This system is used during extended exchanges, aggressive flurries, and trading punches at a high work rate.

The downside? This system produces lactic acid as a byproduct, which causes that burning sensation in the muscles. If not trained properly, fighters will fatigue quickly and struggle to keep up the pace.

Why It's Important in Boxing:

- Fuels fast-paced exchanges and extended combinations.

- Helps fighters maintain a high output of punches without fatiguing too quickly.

- Conditions the body to flush lactic acid faster, delaying muscle fatigue.

How to Train the Anaerobic Lactic System:

- Interval Sprints – 200m or 400m sprints with 45-60 second rest between each rep.

- Heavy Bag Power Rounds – 30-45 second bursts of all-out power punches, followed by short rest.

- High-Intensity Circuit Training – Burpees, medicine ball slams, and battle ropes (work: 45 seconds, rest: 30 seconds).

Common Mistakes:

- Training too long at high intensity—fighters should aim for short, high-power bursts instead of prolonged efforts.

- Ignoring active recovery—cool downs, stretching, and mobility work are needed to prevent overuse injuries.

- Skipping lactic threshold training—fighters need to gradually build their tolerance to fatigue.

When the Anaerobic Lactic System Fails:

If a fighter lacks conditioning in this system, they'll struggle to throw high-volume combinations without gassing out. They might start a flurry strong but then lose power and speed after a few punches.

3. The Anaerobic Alactic Energy System (Explosive Power)

What it Does:

The anaerobic alactic system provides immediate bursts of energy for maximal efforts lasting up to 10 seconds. This system is used when a fighter:

- Throws a knockout punch.

- Explodes out of danger.

- Reacts quickly to an opponent's attack.

Unlike the lactic system, the alactic system doesn't produce fatigue-inducing byproducts. However, it burns out quickly, meaning fighters must have fast recovery to repeatedly use it throughout a fight.

Why it's Important in Boxing:

- Enables quick, explosive power punches.
- Helps fighters evade attacks with rapid movement.
- Improves reaction time and reflexes.

How to Train the Anaerobic Alactic System:

- Short Sprints (20-30m max effort) – Rest fully between reps.
- Olympic Lifts (Power Cleans, Snatches) – Develops explosive muscle contractions.
- Plyometric Training (Jump Squats, Hurdle Jumps, Medicine Ball Slams) – Builds fast-twitch muscle fibers.

Common Mistakes:

- Not allowing full recovery between sets— fighters must rest adequately to train this system properly.
- Ignoring strength training—maximal power requires strong muscles.
- Overdoing long-duration workouts—this system is about short, explosive power, not endurance.

When the Anaerobic Alactic System Fails

A fighter lacking this system will lack knockout power, struggle with explosive movements, and be slow in counter punching or evasion.

Building a Balanced Energy System Training Plan

Since all three systems play a role in boxing, training must be balanced. Here's how to structure a complete energy system plan:

Energy System	Training Focus	Best Methods	Rest Between Sets
Aerobic (Endurance)	Long-duration stamina	Roadwork, jump rope, shadowboxing	Short rest (active recovery)
Anaerobic Lactic (High-Pace Work)	Short-burst high-output	Sprint intervals, high-intensity circuits, bag drills	Moderate rest (45-90 seconds)
Anaerobic Alactic (Explosive Power)	Max-power bursts	Plyometrics, Olympic lifts, short sprints	Full recovery (2-4 min)

Key Takeaways:

- Fighters need all three systems to perform at their best.

- Training must be structured properly—overemphasizing one system can hurt performance.

- Recovery is just as important as training—fatigued fighters don't improve.

Strength training BEFORE camp ensures that fighters don't lose power as weight cutting intensifies later.

CHAPTER 4
Pre-Camp:
Laying the Foundation for
Fight Preparation

Before a fighter begins a full boxing training camp, there's a crucial pre-camp phase that sets the foundation for a successful fight camp. Many fighters make the mistake of jumping straight into high-intensity training without first preparing their body, which leads to burnout, injuries, and inefficient training cycles.

In this chapter, we'll cover:

- The purpose of pre-camp and why it's essential.

- How to test and evaluate a fighter's conditioning before training begins.

- The key training areas to focus on during pre-camp.

- A sample pre-camp training schedule for fighters.

By following a structured pre-camp process, fighters and coaches ensure that when fight camp officially starts, the body is already primed and ready.

What is Pre-Camp and Why is it Important?

Pre-camp is the four to eight week phase before an official training camp begins. It is NOT about peaking for a fight—it's about building the physical foundation necessary for intense boxing-specific training.

Many fighters who neglect pre-camp show up to training camp:

- Out of shape

- Overweight

- Carrying injuries

- Lacking strength and endurance

This wastes valuable time during camp, forcing coaches to spend the first few weeks getting the fighter into basic shape instead of focusing on fight-specific skills.

Pre-Camp Goals:

- Improve base conditioning (endurance, strength, mobility).

- Correct weaknesses and imbalances before high-intensity work begins.

- Prevent early injuries caused by sudden intense training.

Establish good weight management to avoid extreme weight cuts later.

Step 1: Testing and Evaluating a Fighter's Condition

Before designing a pre-camp plan, a full assessment of the fighter's current physical state is necessary. This helps identify weaknesses and determine where the focus should be.

1. Cardiovascular Testing (Heart Rate & Endurance)

A fighter's **heart rate** is one of the best indicators of conditioning. A well-conditioned fighter has:

- A lower resting heart rate (50-60 bpm).
- A faster recovery rate after intense activity.

Tests to Evaluate Cardiovascular Fitness

Heart Rate Recovery Test – Measure heart rate after 1 minute of rest following max effort work.

Three Minute Step Test – Step up and down on a bench for 3 minutes, then measure how fast the heart rate drops.

Twelve Minute Run Test – Measures aerobic endurance and VO2 max.

2. Strength & Power Testing

Strength and power determine how effectively a fighter can generate force in punches, movement, and defensive actions.

Key Tests for Strength & Power:

- Medicine Ball Punch Throws – Tests upper body explosiveness.

- Trap Bar Deadlift 1RM – Measures overall strength and force production.

- Vertical Jump Test – Tests lower-body explosiveness for movement and reaction time.

3. Speed & Agility Testing

Boxing requires quick footwork, explosive movement, and rapid directional changes.

Tests to Evaluate Speed & Agility

10m Sprint Test – Measures initial acceleration.

Ladder Drills & Cone Drills – Tests footwork speed and agility.

Reaction Time Test – Measures reflexes and defensive reaction speed.

4. Mobility & Injury Risk Assessment

Many fighters ignore mobility, which can lead to stiffness, poor movement, and injuries.

Key Mobility Tests

Overhead Squat Test – Assesses flexibility and posture.

Hip Flexor & Hamstring Test – Identifies tightness that can affect movement.

Shoulder Mobility Test – Ensures optimal punching mechanics.

Once these tests are completed, coaches can design a pre-camp plan that focuses on the fighter's weaknesses.

Step 2: Key Training Areas for Pre-Camp

Pre-camp should focus on general fitness and athleticism, NOT full-intensity boxing training. This phase builds a strong foundation so that when camp begins, the fighter can handle high-intensity training.

1. Building a Strong Cardiovascular Base

Boxing is an endurance-based sport, so fighters must have a strong aerobic and anaerobic base.

Pre-Camp Cardio Training:

- Roadwork (3-5 miles, steady pace, 3x per week)- Builds aerobic endurance.

- Interval Sprints (100m sprints, 30 second rest, repeat 10x) – Develops fight-specific conditioning.

- Jump Rope (15-20 minutes per session) – Improves footwork and conditioning.

Why? Building endurance BEFORE fight camp allows for higher-intensity boxing drills later.

2. Strength & Power Development

Many fighters enter camp without adequate strength, which affects their ability to generate explosive punches, maintain posture, and absorb impact.

Pre-Camp Strength Training:

- Squats & Deadlifts – Build overall strength and power.

- Medicine Ball Slams & Throws – Develop explosive punching power.

- Pull-Ups & Push-Ups – Improve upper-body strength for clinching and punching endurance.

Why? Strength training BEFORE camp ensures that fighters don't lose power as weight cutting intensifies later.

3. Speed & Agility Work

Footwork is essential in boxing, and pre-camp is the best time to improve quickness, movement efficiency, and reflexes.

Pre-Camp Speed & Agility Drills:

- Ladder Drills (3x per week) – Improves foot speed and coordination.

- Reaction Drills (Coach Calls or Flash Reflex Training) – Enhances fight reflexes.

- Bounding & Plyometrics – Improves explosive movement in and out of exchanges.

Why? Fast, agile fighters control the ring and avoid damage better than slow, flat-footed fighters.

4. Mobility & Injury Prevention

Many fighters neglect flexibility and joint mobility, leading to poor movement and increased risk of injury.

Pre-Camp Mobility Routine:

- Dynamic Stretching (Before Training) – Loosens muscles for better movement.

- Foam Rolling & Myofascial Release – Prevents stiffness and aids recovery.

- Yoga or Controlled Flexibility Work (1-2x per week) – Improves range of motion.

Why? Improved mobility enhances movement efficiency and reduces injury risk.

Step 3: Sample 4-Week Pre-Camp Training Schedule

A fighter's pre-camp schedule should include a mix of cardio, strength, speed, and mobility training to prepare for intense fight camp work.

Day	Training Focus
Monday	Strength (Squats, Pull-Ups, Medicine Ball Slams) + Jump Rope (15 mins)
Tuesday	Roadwork (3 miles) + Agility Ladder Drills + Mobility Work
Wednesday	Interval Sprints (10x100m) + Boxing Drills (Light Sparring)
Thursday	Strength (Deadlifts, Push-Ups, Core Work) + Jump Rope
Friday	Speed & Footwork Drills + Reaction Training
Saturday	Active Recovery (Swimming, Mobility, Stretching)
Sunday	Rest / Recovery

This schedule gradually increases intensity, so when fight camp starts, the fighter is already in shape and ready for serious boxing-specific training.

Conclusion: Pre-Camp is the Key to a Strong Fight Camp

A fighter who enters camp in peak shape has a massive advantage over opponents who spend camp just trying to get fit. Pre-camp builds the foundation so that every second of training camp can focus on boxing skills, fight strategy, and sharpening tools.

- Pre-camp prevents injuries, improves conditioning, and enhances overall performance.

- Testing before pre-camp helps coaches design a personalized training approach.

- A structured pre-camp program ensures fighters are physically ready for intense training.

A properly executed 8-week training camp ensures that a fighter enters the ring strong, explosive, and prepared for all 12 rounds.

CHAPTER 5

Training Camp: The 8-Week Plan for Fight Night

Once pre-camp is complete and a fighter enters training camp, the focus shifts from building a foundation to fight-specific preparation. This is the most intense phase of a fighter's training cycle, designed to maximize strength, endurance, speed, and technical sharpness before stepping into the ring.

In this chapter, we'll break down:

- The purpose and structure of an 8-week training camp.

- How to balance boxing skills, strength, and conditioning without over training.

- A week-by-week breakdown of how fighters should train leading up to fight night.

- How to peak at the right time for optimal performance on fight night.

A well-structured training camp ensures that a fighter steps into the ring in peak condition, both physically and mentally.

What Happens During an 8-Week Training Camp?

Training camp is not about getting in shape—that should have been done in pre-camp. Instead, this phase is about:

- Sharpening boxing skills

- Building fight-specific endurance

- Maximizing explosive power and speed

- Fine-tuning weight and recovery strategies

- Developing a game plan for the opponent

A properly planned camp prevents:

- Over training – Too much volume and intensity can lead to fatigue, decreased performance, or injuries.

- Under training – If a fighter is not pushed hard enough, they won't be physically prepared for fight night.

- Poor weight management – Extreme weight cuts or bad nutrition choices can ruin performance.

Balancing Strength, Conditioning, and Boxing Training

Many coaches struggle with how to balance strength & conditioning with boxing training. The key is to:

1. Prioritize skill work – Boxing training (sparring, bag work, mitts) should always come first.

2. Use strength & conditioning to enhance boxing performance – Avoid training like a bodybuilder or marathon runner.

3. Monitor fatigue levels – Fighters should train hard but recover properly to avoid burnout.

Training Breakdown:

- Boxing Skills (60-70% of total training)- Includes sparring, pad work, bag drills, footwork, and technical drills.

- Strength & Conditioning (30-40% of total training) – Includes strength training, explosive power, agility, and endurance work.

- Recovery & Mobility (Daily focus) – Includes stretching, massage, ice baths, and sleep optimization.

Week-By-Week Breakdown of an 8-Week Training Camp

Weeks 1-2: Building Fight-Ready Conditioning

- **Focus:** Base conditioning, volume work, and strength maintenance.

- **Boxing Training:** High volume, technical drilling, moderate sparring.

- **Strength & Conditioning:** Full-body strength training, endurance work, footwork drills.

SAMPLE WEEKLY SCHEDULE

Day	Boxing Work	Strength & Conditioning
Monday	Technical drills, bag work	Full-body strength (squats, deadlifts, pull-ups)
Tuesday	Heavy bag, footwork drills	Sprint intervals (200m, 400m)
Wednesday	Pad work, light sparring	Explosive training (medicine ball throws, plyometrics)
Thursday	Shadowboxing, mitts	Strength training (upper body focus)
Friday	Heavy bag, sparring	Agility ladder, reaction drills
Saturday	Light drills, strategy work	Recovery (mobility, stretching, ice baths)
Sunday	Rest	Recovery

- Sparring should be light-to-moderate volume to avoid early injuries.

- Strength training should maintain power without causing excessive fatigue.

- Focus on mobility and flexibility to prevent early stiffness.

Weeks 3-4: Increasing Intensity & Power

- **Focus:** Sharpening boxing skills, increasing power and explosiveness.

- **Boxing Training:** Sparring intensity increases, pad work gets sharper.

- **Strength & Conditioning:** Explosive power movements, short sprint work.

Key Adjustments:

- Sparring increases to 2-3 times per week.

- Strength training focuses on explosive movements (trap bar deadlifts, medicine ball throws).

- Conditioning includes short, intense sprint work.

Weeks 5-6: Peak Training Phase (Hardest Workload)

- **Focus:** Maximizing speed, power, and endurance for fight conditions.

- **Boxing Training:** High-volume sparring (8-12 rounds), intense mitt work.

- **Strength & Conditioning:** Sport-specific drills, maintaining peak explosiveness.

Key Adjustments:

- Sparring intensity at its highest (simulating fight pace).

- Strength training shifts to maintenance mode (no heavy lifting).

- Conditioning focuses on short, explosive bursts to mimic fight intensity.

- Watch for signs of overtraining (excessive fatigue, poor recovery, mood swings).

- Nutrition and hydration must be optimized to prepare for weight cut.

Weeks 7-8: Tapering & Peaking for Fight Night

- **Focus:** Speed, timing, and fight readiness—reducing training volume to avoid burnout.

- **Boxing Training:** Lighter sparring, precision work, focusing on fight strategy.

- **Strength & Conditioning:** Speed and agility drills, active recovery work.

Key Adjustments:

- Sparring tapers down to avoid unnecessary damage.

- Weight-cutting strategy is in place to make weight safely.

- Emphasis on sleep, hydration, and recovery.

- By the end of Week 8, the fighter should feel sharp, explosive, and fully recovered.

Peaking for Fight Night: The Final 7 Days

The last week is all about timing, recovery, and mental preparation.

DAY	FOCUS
Monday	Light drills, final strength session (low volume)
Tuesday	Speed drills, reaction training
Wednesday	Last technical session, stretching & mobility
Thursday	Light mitt work, tapering down
Friday	Rest, making weight, hydration protocol
Saturday (Fight Night)	Fully recovered, peak performance

- Hydration and weight-cutting are closely monitored to avoid extreme depletion.

- Mental focus is a priority—visualization, relaxation, and strategy discussions.

- No excessive training—fighter must enter fight night fresh and sharp.

The Keys to a Successful Training Camp

To ensure a fighter peaks perfectly on fight night, follow these principles:

- Boxing skills come first – Strength & conditioning supports boxing, not the other way around.

- Strength and conditioning must be balanced – Avoid overtraining, keep sessions efficient.

- Monitor fatigue and recovery – Use heart rate tracking, sleep monitoring, and nutrition adjustments.

- Taper down before fight night – Fighters should arrive fresh, not overworked.

- Weight cutting must be strategic – Fighters should not be cutting excessive weight in the final days.

A properly executed 8-week training camp ensures that a fighter enters the ring strong, explosive, and prepared for all 12 rounds.

A successful weight cut can be the difference between winning and losing on fight night.

CHAPTER 6
Weight Cutting and Fight Week Nutrition

Weight cutting is one of the most critical and dangerous aspects of boxing. A poorly executed weight cut can drain energy, reduce performance, and even put a fighter's health at risk. On the other hand, a smart and strategic weight cut can ensure that a fighter makes weight without sacrificing strength, endurance, or recovery.

In this chapter, we'll cover:

- The science of weight cutting and why it must be done correctly.

- The dangers of extreme dehydration and how to prevent it.

- A week-by-week breakdown of weight management before the fight.

- How to rehydrate and refuel after weigh-ins for maximum performance.

A successful weight cut can be the difference between winning and losing on fight night.

Understanding Weight Cutting: The Right Way vs. The Wrong Way

Many fighters cut weight the wrong way, relying on starvation, extreme dehydration, and last-minute sauna sessions to shed pounds. This is dangerous and can lead to:

- Muscle loss – Weakens punches and endurance.

- Severe dehydration – Increases risk of brain injury and slows reaction time.

- Reduced endurance – A dehydrated fighter fatigues faster.

- Poor recovery – Lack of nutrients prevents peak performance.

How Weight Cutting Works

A proper weight cut happens in **t**wo phases:

1. Long-Term Weight Management (8-4 weeks out) – Gradually reducing body fat while maintaining muscle and energy.

2. Short-Term Water Manipulation (Seven days before weigh-in) – Temporarily reducing water weight without harming performance.

Key Rule: Never cut more than 5-7% of body weight in the final week. Anything more will significantly damage performance.

Weeks 8-4: Long-Term Weight Management

The best fighters don't wait until the last minute to cut weight. They maintain a fight-ready physique year-round, making the final cut much easier.

Goals During This Phase:

- Maintain muscle mass while gradually lowering body fat.

- Reduce unnecessary water retention (limit sodium, avoid processed foods).

- Increase protein intake to preserve strength.

- Control carbohydrate intake (not eliminate, just regulate).

Best Foods for Long-Term Weight Management:

- Lean Proteins – Chicken, fish, turkey, lean beef, eggs.

- Complex Carbohydrates (moderate amounts) – Brown rice, quinoa, oatmeal, sweet potatoes.

- Healthy Fats – Avocados, nuts, olive oil, salmon.

- Vegetables & High-Fiber Foods – Help digestion and reduce bloating.

- Plenty of Water – Hydration is key for maintaining metabolism.

Foods to Avoid:

- High-Sodium Foods – Causes water retention and bloating.

- Processed Junk Food – Adds unnecessary fat and weight.

- Excess Sugars & Artificial Sweeteners – Disrupts energy levels and hydration balance.

Final Seven Days: Safe Water Manipulation for Weigh-Ins

The final week before weigh-ins is where temporary water weight reduction is used to make weight without damaging performance.

Day	Water Intake	Sodium Intake	Carb Intake
7 Days Out	1 gallons	Normal	Normal
6 Days Out	1 gallons	Reduced	Low
5 Days Out	.75 gallons	Reduced	Low
4 Days Out	.75 gallons	Low	Very Low
3 Days Out	1.75 gallon	Very Low	Very Low
2 Days Out	0.5 gallon	No sodium	No carbs
1 Day Before Weigh-In	0.5 gallon	No sodium	No carbs

Why This Works:

- Drinking extra water tricks the body into flushing out excess water.

- Reducing sodium prevents bloating and unnecessary water retention.

- Lowering carbohydrates removes stored glycogen, reducing weight.

- The fighter enters the weigh-in dehydrated, but safely.

The Final 24 Hours: Cutting the Last Few Pounds

If a fighter is still over the weight limit the day before weigh-ins, they can safely cut 1-3 more pounds using:

- Sauna or Hot Baths – Sweat out final water weight (15 minutes in, 5 minutes out).

- Light Cardio (Sweat Suit Workouts) – Only if needed, light movement to lose water weight.

- No solid food until after weigh-in.

- Never cut too much water weight. If a fighter needs to lose more than 5-7% of their body weight in the final week, they mismanaged their weight earlier.

Post-Weigh-In:
Rehydration & Refueling for Fight Night

Once the weigh-in is over, refueling properly is critical to restore energy, endurance, and strength.

First 30 Minutes After Weigh-In:

- 16-20 oz electrolyte drink (Pedialyte, coconut water, sports drink).

- Small, easy-to-digest meal (Banana, oats, honey, almond butter).

Next 2-4 Hours:

- Reintroduce carbohydrates (Rice, potatoes, fruit).

- More lean protein (Chicken, fish, eggs).

- Hydrate continuously (Avoid drinking too fast to prevent bloating).

Final Pre-Fight Meal (4-6 Hours Before Fight):

- Balanced meal with carbs, protein, and healthy fats.

- Avoid heavy, greasy, or slow-digesting foods.

- Drink water consistently but do not over hydrate.

Common Mistakes in Weight Cutting

- Cutting weight too aggressively – Leads to extreme fatigue and poor performance.

- Skipping meals to lose weight faster – Causes muscle loss and weakness.

- Not rehydrating properly after weigh-ins – Leads to sluggishness and poor endurance.

- Relying on extreme sauna or sweat suit sessions – Increases risk of dehydration and brain damage.

The Smart Way to Make Weight

A well-planned weight cut ensures that a fighter:

- Makes weight safely without losing power.

- Enters the ring fully fueled and hydrated.

- Maintains endurance, strength, and sharpness.

- Avoids unnecessary health risks from extreme dehydration.

By following long-term weight management strategies and using smart water manipulation, fighters can make weight effectively while staying strong and explosive.

A strong, durable, and well-recovered fighter is a dangerous fighter.

CHAPTER 7
Recovery and Injury Prevention in Boxing

Boxing is one of the most physically demanding sports in the world. Fighters push their bodies to the limit with intense training, sparring, and competition. However, without proper recovery and injury prevention strategies, a fighter's career can be cut short due to overtraining, chronic injuries, or burnout.

In this chapter, we'll cover:

- The importance of recovery in boxing

- How to prevent common injuries

- Best recovery techniques for faster healing

- How strength & conditioning can extend a fighter's career

A strong, durable, and well-recovered fighter is a dangerous fighter.

Why Recovery is Critical for Fighters

Many fighters believe that more training is always better, but this is a mistake. Recovery is just as important as training because:

- Muscles grow and repair during rest, not during training.
- Overtraining leads to fatigue, decreased performance, and injuries.
- A well-recovered fighter is stronger, sharper, and more explosive.

Fighters who ignore recovery often experience:

- Chronic injuries (shoulder, knee, back pain).
- Overtraining symptoms (fatigue, mood swings, slow reaction time).
- Inconsistent performances due to exhaustion.
- Proper recovery ensures that fighters perform at their best on fight night.

Common Injuries in Boxing and How to Prevent Them

Boxing puts immense stress on the body. Here are the most common injuries and how to prevent them:

1. Hand & Wrist Injuries

Cause: Repetitive impact from punching, poor hand wrapping, improper punching technique.

Prevention:

- Always wrap hands properly before training.
- Use properly padded gloves for heavy bag work.
- Strengthen wrist and forearm muscles with grip exercises & wrist rolls.

2. Shoulder Injuries (Rotator Cuff, Impingement)

Cause: Overuse from excessive punching, weak stabilizing muscles.

Prevention:

- Strengthen rotator cuff with band exercises & shoulder mobility work.
- Balance training with pulling exercises (rows, pull-ups) to prevent imbalances.
- Avoid overuse—limit excessive bag work to prevent strain.

3. Concussions & Head Trauma

Cause: Repeated blows to the head, improper defensive skills.

Prevention:

- Prioritize head movement, blocking, and defensive drills.
- Reduce hard sparring to avoid unnecessary

head trauma.

- Strengthen the neck muscles to absorb impact.

4. Knee & Ankle Injuries

Cause: Poor footwork mechanics, lack of mobility, weak stabilizer muscles.

Prevention:

- Strengthen hips, glutes, and lower leg muscles for joint stability.

- Improve footwork technique to avoid awkward movements.

- Do mobility exercises for ankle and knee flexibility.

5. Lower Back Pain & Core Weakness

Cause: Weak core, poor posture, overuse in twisting motions.

Prevention:

- Strengthen the core with planks, rotational exercises, and stability drills.

- Improve hip mobility to reduce strain on the lower back.

- Use proper posture when throwing punches.

Best Recovery Techniques for Fighters

A fighter's recovery plan is just as important as their training plan. The best fighters recover smarter, allowing them to train harder while avoiding injuries.

1. Sleep: The #1 Recovery Tool

- Fighters should get 7-9 hours of quality sleep per night.
- Sleep is when muscles repair, the nervous system recovers, and hormones regulate.
- Use cool, dark, quiet environments to optimize sleep quality.

2. Nutrition & Hydration for Faster Recovery

- Eat high-protein meals to rebuild muscle tissue.
- Replenish glycogen with complex carbs after training.
- Stay hydrated—even 2% dehydration reduces performance.
- Include anti-inflammatory foods (salmon, turmeric, blueberries) to speed up healing.

3. Active Recovery (Light Movement & Stretching)

After intense training, light movement helps flush out lactic acid and promotes blood flow.

- Foam rolling & mobility drills to improve flexibility.

- Low-intensity shadowboxing to loosen muscles.

- Swimming or cycling for low-impact recovery sessions.

4. Ice Baths & Heat Therapy

- Ice baths reduce inflammation and muscle soreness after heavy training.

- Heat therapy (saunas, hot baths) promotes blood flow and muscle relaxation.

5. Massage & Physical Therapy

- Deep tissue massage breaks up muscle knots and improves circulation.

- Sports chiropractic care realigns the spine and improves mobility.

- Active Release Therapy (ART) reduces scar tissue and improves flexibility.

6. Breathing & Relaxation Techniques

- Deep breathing exercises reduce stress and improve recovery.

- Meditation or mindfulness helps fighters stay calm and focused.

- Controlled nasal breathing improves oxygen efficiency in the ring.

How Strength & Conditioning Prevents Injuries

A proper strength and conditioning program is the best way to prevent injuries and extend a fighter's career.

- Strengthens muscles, tendons, and ligaments, reducing stress on joints.

- Improves mobility and flexibility, preventing stiffness and overuse injuries.

- Corrects muscular imbalances, ensuring the body functions efficiently.

- Enhances core stability, improving punch mechanics and balance.

Key Strength Exercises for Injury Prevention

- Deadlifts & Squats – Build total-body strength and joint stability.

- Pull-Ups & Rows – Strengthen the upper back and prevent shoulder injuries.

- Core Rotation Drills – Improve punch power and protect the lower back.

- Hip & Glute Strengthening – Reduce knee and ankle stress.

Overtraining: When More Training Becomes a Problem

Some fighters train too much and recover too little, leading to over training syndrome. Signs of overtraining include:

Chronic fatigue (feeling drained even after rest).

Loss of speed and power (punches feel slower and weaker).

Increased injuries (body is constantly sore and in pain).

Mental burnout (lack of motivation, mood swings, depression).

How to Avoid Overtraining:

- Listen to the body—train hard but recover harder.

- Monitor heart rate & fatigue levels (high resting heart rate = possible overtraining).

- Take de-load weeks (reduce intensity every 4-6 weeks to allow recovery).

- Prioritize sleep, nutrition, and stress management.

The Key to Longevity in Boxing

A fighter's career can be short or long, depending on how well they train, recover, and prevent injuries. Fighters who take care of their bodies last longer, perform better, and avoid career-ending injuries.

- Train smart, not just hard—balance volume and intensity.

- Prioritize recovery—it's just as important as training.

- Strength train properly to avoid common injuries.

- Listen to the body—rest when needed to prevent burnout.

- Use proper nutrition, hydration, and sleep to stay in peak condition.

Proper recovery ensures that fighters perform at their best on fight night.

CHAPTER 8

Mental Toughness & Psychology for Boxing

Boxing is often called the "sweet science," but beyond the physical training, strength, and endurance, one of the biggest factors in a fighter's success is mental toughness. Many great fighters have lost fights not because they lacked skill, but because they lacked mental fortitude. On the other hand, fighters with ironclad mental strength have overcome adversity, fatigue, and tough opponents to become world champions.

In this chapter, we'll cover:

- Why mental toughness is just as important as physical strength.

- The key psychological traits of elite fighters.

- How to develop confidence, focus, and resilience.

- Techniques to stay calm under pressure and perform at your best on fight night.

Boxing is not just about throwing punches—it's about staying composed, strategic, and mentally unbreakable under extreme stress.

The Importance of Mental Toughness in Boxing

A fighter can be in peak physical condition, but if they mentally break under pressure, doubt themselves, or hesitate in the ring, they will lose. Mental toughness determines:

- How a fighter handles pressure and adversity.
- Whether they can keep going when exhausted.
- How well they stick to a game plan.
- Their ability to stay composed when hurt or frustrated.

Examples of Mental Toughness in Boxing:

- Muhammad Ali – Overcame extreme adversity in fights, stayed calm under pressure, and used psychological tactics to gain an edge.
- Floyd Mayweather Jr. – Maintained laser-sharp focus, never let emotions dictate his game plan, and never lost control.
- Mike Tyson – Fought with ruthless aggression and self-belief, intimidating opponents before the fight even started.
- Tyson Fury – Got knocked down by Deontay Wilder but mentally refused to lose, rising from the canvas and fighting back.

A physically tough fighter without mental toughness

will break. A mentally strong fighter will keep fighting no matter what.

Key Psychological Traits of Elite Fighters

1. Confidence: Believing You Will Win

Self-belief is the foundation of success in boxing. If a fighter doubts themselves, they are already at a disadvantage.

- Confident fighters fight smarter, commit to their punches, and take risks when needed.

- They trust their training, don't hesitate, and control the pace of the fight.

- Confidence is built through consistent preparation, success in training, and self-discipline.

How to Develop Confidence

- Train like a champion. Confidence comes from preparation—knowing you've put in the work.

- Positive self-talk. Never say "I hope I win"—say "I will win."

- Focus on strengths, not weaknesses. Visualize yourself executing your best moves, not making mistakes.

- *Mistake:* Some fighters gain false confidence

through easy sparring or weak opponents. Real confidence comes from testing yourself under tough conditions.

2. Composure Under Pressure

The ability to stay calm in the ring is what separates great fighters from average ones. Some fighters panic when they get hit, lose control of their emotions, or rush their attacks—this leads to mistakes.

- Calm fighters think clearly, read their opponents, and stick to their game plan.

- They don't waste energy by fighting with emotions.

- They stay composed, even when things aren't going their way.

How to Stay Calm Under Pressure

Controlled breathing: Slow, deep breaths reduce adrenaline overload.

Mental rehearsals: Visualize yourself remaining composed during tough moments.

Training in high-pressure situations: Hard sparring, fighting while tired, and simulating fight-night conditions.

Mistake: Some fighters lose focus and start brawling when they feel pressured—this plays into the opponent's game.

3. Resilience & Grit: The Ability to Keep Fighting

A champion mindset means never giving up, no matter what. Fighters with true grit keep pushing through pain, fatigue, and adversity.

- Resilient fighters don't make excuses or quit when things get tough.

- They push through exhaustion in the later rounds.

- They embrace suffering in training, knowing it prepares them for war.

How to Build Resilience

Train through discomfort. Do extra rounds when tired.

Develop a strong "why." Understand why you fight—this fuels determination.

Learn from failures. Champions don't let losses break them; they use them to improve.

Mistake: Some fighters make excuses or blame external factors instead of taking responsibility for their improvement.

4. Focus & Fight IQ: Thinking Like a Champion

Boxing is not just physical—it's a chess match. The best fighters are thinking fighters who analyze, adapt, and stay focused throughout the fight.

- Focused fighters read their opponents, adjust strategies, and stay one step ahead.

- They don't get distracted by the crowd, trash talk, or frustration.

- They stay locked in on their game plan and execute it with precision.

How to Improve Focus & Fight IQ

- Study fights: Watch high-level fighters and analyze their tactics.

- Practice mindfulness: Train yourself to block out distractions.

- Spar with a purpose: Instead of just throwing punches, focus on specific strategies.

- *Mistake:* Some fighters lose focus and get emotionally invested in landing one big punch, instead of sticking to their strategy.

Mental Training Techniques for Boxing

Fighters must train their minds just like they train their bodies. Here are the best mental training techniques:

1. Visualization: Seeing Victory Before It Happens

Close your eyes and picture yourself:

- Walking to the ring with confidence.

- Dodging punches and landing clean shots.

- Staying strong and focused in the later rounds.

Why it works: The brain cannot distinguish between real and vividly imagined experiences—this makes visualization a powerful tool for success.

2. Positive Self-Talk: Controlling Your Inner Voice

What a fighter says to themselves matters. Fighters who tell themselves "I'm strong, I'm fast, I'm prepared" perform better than those who think "I'm tired, I'm not ready."

- Use affirmations daily: "I am a warrior. I am ready for battle."

- Eliminate negative thoughts: If you think "I'm too tired," replace it with "I've trained for this."

- *Mistake:* Negative self-talk destroys confidence. Never let doubt control your mind.

3. Controlling Fear & Nerves on Fight Night

Every fighter feels fear and adrenaline before a fight. The key is controlling it and using it to your advantage.

- Deep breathing exercises slow the heart rate and reduce nerves.

- Routine & rituals (warm-ups, pre-fight habits) create familiarity and calmness.

- Reframing fear as excitement helps turn nerves into positive energy.

- *Mistake:* Some fighters burn themselves out by getting too hyped before the fight—this leads to an energy dump in the early rounds.

The Mental Edge: Training Like a Champion

The best fighters train their minds as much as their bodies. Mental toughness is what separates the great from the good.

Confidence, composure, resilience, and focus are all trainable skills.

- Mental preparation must be part of every fighter's routine.

- Champions don't just have strong bodies—they have strong minds.

CHAPTER 9

Developing the Perfect Fight Night Routine

Fight night is where everything comes together—all the training, conditioning, mental preparation, and strategy. However, even the best-prepared fighters can underperform if they don't have a proper fight night routine.

A fighter must be mentally sharp, physically primed, and emotionally controlled when stepping into the ring. A poor warm-up, last-minute nerves, or even a bad pre-fight meal can affect performance.

In this chapter, we'll cover:

- How to create the perfect fight night routine

- The best warm-up strategy for peak performance

- Mental and physical preparation before stepping into the ring

- How to control adrenaline and start the fight strong

Why a Fight Night Routine is Crucial

Many fighters lose before the fight even starts because they make simple mistakes:

- Warming up too much or too little—causing early fatigue or stiffness.

- Getting too nervous or too relaxed—losing focus.

- Overeating or under eating before the fight—leading to sluggishness.

- Not mentally locking in—losing confidence before the first bell.

A structured fight night routine ensures that a fighter enters the ring in peak condition—physically and mentally.

Fight Night Preparation: The Final 24 Hours

1. The Pre-Fight Meal (4-6 Hours Before the Fight)

- Balanced meal with carbs, protein, and healthy fats for sustained energy.

- Drink water consistently—not too much at once to avoid bloating.

Avoid heavy, greasy, or slow-digesting foods that can cause sluggishness.

Best Pre-Fight Meal Examples:

- Option 1: Grilled chicken, brown rice, steamed vegetables.

- Option 2: Salmon, sweet potatoes, avocado.

- Option 3: Oatmeal, banana, almond butter.

Avoid caffeine and energy drinks late in the day— they can cause an energy crash later.

2. The Mental Routine: Locking Into Fight Mode

- Visualization exercises—mentally rehearse the fight, see yourself winning.

- Positive self-talk—use affirmations like "I am ready, I am powerful, I am unstoppable."

- Stay off your phone—limit distractions and social media.

- Champions like Floyd Mayweather and Tyson Fury use mental routines to stay focused before stepping into the ring.

Avoid getting too hyped too early—conserve energy for the fight.

The Pre-Fight Warm-Up
(30-45 Minutes Before Fight Time)

How to Warm Up for Maximum Performance

The warm-up must:

- Activate the muscles for speed and power.

- Get the heart rate up without over-fatiguing the body.

- Sharpen reaction time and mental focus.

Ideal Warm-Up Routine
(30-45 Minutes Before Fight Time)

Time	Activity	Purpose
0-5 Min	Light jogging & dynamic stretching	Loosens muscles, increases blood flow
5-10 Min	Shadowboxing (gradually increasing intensity)	Warms up movement, sharpens reflexes
10-20 Min	Mitt work (short rounds, fast hands)	Improves reaction time, timing, and coordination
20-30 Min	Footwork drills & defensive movement	Prepares legs for ring movement
30-35 Min	Explosive plyometrics (short jumps, fast punches)	Activates fast-twitch muscles
35-40 Min	Light breathing exercises & final mindset prep	Controls nerves, locks in focus

Common Warm-Up Mistakes:

- Warming up too hard—wasting energy before the fight.

- Not warming up enough—leading to slow starts and stiffness.

- Skipping mental preparation—causing hesitation and poor confidence.

Walking to the Ring:
How to Control Adrenaline & Nerves

Even the greatest fighters feel nerves before stepping into the ring. The key is controlling the adrenaline rush so that it enhances performance instead of causing panic.

- Control your breathing. Slow, deep breaths calm the nervous system.

- Keep a calm but confident mindset. Avoid overthinking.

- Stick to the game plan. Remind yourself of the strategy.

- Embrace the moment. Use the energy of the crowd as fuel.

- **Example:** Mike Tyson used to repeat to himself, *"I am the best. I am the greatest. No one can stop me."*

- *Mistake:* Some fighters let adrenaline overwhelm them and start too fast, burning out in the early rounds.

Starting the Fight: Setting the Tone in Round One

How a fighter starts the first round can dictate the entire fight.

Establish dominance early—control the center of the ring.

Stay relaxed but focused—don't rush into reckless exchanges.

Read your opponent—assess their speed, reactions, and movement.

Use feints and jabs to create openings.

Great fighters don't waste energy in Round 1—they set traps, control the pace, and break opponents down strategically.

Mistake: Fighters who throw wild punches early often gas out and lose their rhythm.

The Winning Mindset for Fight Night

To win a fight, a fighter must have:

Confidence—knowing they trained harder and are prepared to win.

Composure—staying relaxed and making smart decisions.

Adaptability—adjusting to the opponent's style and weaknesses.

Relentlessness—pushing through fatigue, pain, and adversity.

A fighter's mindset on fight night determines whether they rise to the occasion or crumble under pressure.

Final Checklist for Fight Night Success

Pre-Fight Routine (4-6 Hours Before)

- Eat a balanced pre-fight meal
- Stay hydrated (but don't over drink)
- Do mental visualization and self-talk
- Avoid distractions and social media

Warm-Up (30-45 Minutes Before)

- Activate muscles with movement drills
- Sharpen reflexes with mitt work & shadowboxing Stay loose but mentally locked in

Walking to the Ring

- Control breathing and stay composed
- Focus on the game plan, not emotions
- Embrace the moment and fight with confidence

Round One Strategy

- Establish control of the ring

- Read the opponent's movements and weaknesses

- Stay relaxed but alert—don't waste energy

Conclusion: The Blueprint for Fight Night Success

A fighter with a structured fight night routine steps into the ring:

Physically ready—properly warmed up and activated.

Mentally focused—calm, confident, and locked in.

Emotionally controlled—not letting nerves or adrenaline affect performance.

CHAPTER 10

The Champion's Lifestyle: Training, Nutrition & Recovery Year-Round

The difference between a good fighter and a great fighter isn't just what happens in training camp—it's about how they live every day. True champions don't just train hard for a fight; they live a lifestyle that supports peak performance year-round.

This chapter will cover:

- How elite fighters train, eat, and recover even when they're not in fight camp.

- Why maintaining discipline between fights is crucial for longevity.

- The daily habits that separate champions from average fighters.

Winning starts long before fight night—it starts with the lifestyle a fighter chooses every day.

Why Training Year-Round is Essential

Many fighters make the mistake of only training hard when they have a fight scheduled. This leads to:

- Gaining too much weight between fights.

- Losing conditioning and having to start over every camp.

- Higher risk of injuries due to inconsistent training.

- Shorter careers because of poor long-term habits.

The Champion's Mindset: Always Stay Ready

- Champions don't have to "get in shape" for camp because they stay in shape year-round.

- They never let their weight get out of control.

- They train regularly even when they don't have a fight scheduled.

- They maintain proper recovery, nutrition, and strength work to extend their careers.

Example: Floyd Mayweather stayed in the gym year-round. Even without a fight booked, he was always staying sharp, training, and keeping his weight in check.

Training Year-Round: The Off-Season Blueprint

When a fighter is not in a fight camp, their training should focus on maintaining skills, strength, and endurance without over training.

Off-Season Training Schedule (When No Fight is Scheduled)

Day	Training Focus
Monday	Strength & conditioning (full-body) + light bag work
Tuesday	Boxing drills (mitts, footwork, shadow-boxing) + core work
Wednesday	Sprint intervals + explosive strength training
Thursday	Technical sparring + endurance work (jump rope, roadwork)
Friday	Strength & power training + light bag work
Saturday	Active recovery (swimming, stretching, yoga)
Sunday	Rest or light movement drills

Key Focuses in the Off-Season

Skill sharpening – Work on technique without the pressure of a fight.

Strength maintenance – Stay strong without over training.

Weight control – Keep body weight within 5-10 lbs of fight weight.

Recovery & injury prevention – Focus on joint health and flexibility.

Mistake: Some fighters stop training completely after a fight and gain 20-30 lbs, making it harder to get back in shape for their next camp.

Nutrition for Year-Round Peak Performance

A fighter's diet isn't just for fight camp—it's a lifestyle. Eating the right foods consistently ensures:

- Faster recovery from training.

- Better endurance and strength.

- Optimal brain function and reaction time.

- Easier weight management before a fight.

The Champion's Daily Diet

Protein for muscle recovery – Lean meats, fish, eggs, plant-based protein.

Complex carbs for energy – Brown rice, quinoa, sweet potatoes, oats.

Healthy fats for brain function – Avocados, nuts, olive oil, salmon.

Hydration for performance – At least 1 gallon of water per day.

Vegetables & fruit for vitamins and minerals – Dark leafy greens, berries, bananas.

Ideal Fighter's Daily Meal Plan:

- Breakfast: Scrambled eggs, avocado, whole-grain toast, berries.

- Lunch: Grilled chicken, brown rice, steamed vegetables.

- Snack: Protein shake with banana and almond butter.

- Dinner: Baked salmon, quinoa, roasted sweet potatoes.

- Post-training snack: Greek yogurt with honey and nuts.

Foods to Avoid Year-Round:

- Processed junk food – Causes weight gain and slows recovery.

- Sugary drinks and energy drinks – Lead to energy crashes.

- Fast food and fried food – Increases inflammation and slows muscle recovery.

- Too much alcohol – Affects hydration and muscle repair.

Example: Canelo Álvarez follows a strict, clean diet year-round to maintain his conditioning and prevent drastic weight cuts.

Recovery Habits for Longevity

Many fighters train hard but neglect recovery, leading to injuries and burnout. Proper recovery separates fighters who have long careers from those who burn out early.

Best Recovery Techniques for Fighters

- Sleep – Seven to nine hours per night for muscle repair.

- Hydration – Staying hydrated reduces fatigue and prevents cramps.

- Foam rolling & stretching – Reduces muscle tightness and improves flexibility.

- Cold therapy (ice baths, cryotherapy) – Reduces inflammation after tough workouts.

- Active recovery – Swimming, yoga, or light movement on rest days.

Example: LeBron James and Cristiano Ronaldo invest heavily in recovery strategies—this is why they

perform at an elite level into their late 30s. Fighters must do the same to extend their careers.

Mistake: Some fighters only focus on training but ignore sleep, hydration, and proper recovery, leading to unnecessary injuries.

Mindset: Champions Don't Take Shortcuts

The best fighters don't just train hard—they stay disciplined 24/7.

- They never let themselves get out of shape.

- They treat their body like a machine—fueling it properly.

- They maintain a championship mindset all year long.

- Fighters who only train seriously when a fight is scheduled often struggle with consistency, poor performances, and shorter careers.

Example: Bernard Hopkins fought at an elite level until age 50 because he treated his training, nutrition, and recovery as a lifestyle.

The Blueprint for a Champion's Lifestyle

Daily Habits for Long-Term Success

- Train year-round—never get too far from fight shape.

- Eat clean even when not in fight camp.

- Prioritize sleep, hydration, and recovery.

- Avoid unnecessary weight gain.

- Stay mentally disciplined—act like a champion every day.

Off-Season Training Guidelines

- Train at least 4-5 days per week to maintain strength and skill.

- Work on technical improvements without the pressure of an upcoming fight.

- Keep sparring light and strategic—avoid unnecessary damage.

- Focus on injury prevention and recovery.

Long-Term Nutrition & Health

- Keep weight within 5-10 lbs of fight weight year-round.

- Eat high-protein, nutrient-dense meals daily.

- Avoid excessive junk food and alcohol.

- Stay hydrated and monitor recovery.

Conclusion: Champions Train for Life, Not Just Fights

- A fighter's daily habits and lifestyle determine their longevity, performance, and success.

- Train, eat, and recover like a champion even when no fight is scheduled.

- Avoid weight gain and stay sharp year-round.

Discipline in the off-season leads to dominance in the ring.

CHAPTER 11

The Future of Strength & Conditioning in Boxing

Boxing has always evolved. From bare-knuckle brawls in the 17th century to the scientific training methods of today, the sport continues to change. But what's next?

The future of boxing strength and conditioning is being shaped by:

- Advancements in sports science

- New technology for tracking performance

- Better recovery methods to extend careers

- More specialized training for speed, power, and endurance

In this chapter, we'll explore how boxing training is evolving and what fighters need to do to stay ahead of the competition.

How Sports Science is Changing Boxing

For decades, boxing training was based on tradition and experience rather than science. Fighters relied on:

- Excessive roadwork (long, slow-distance running that doesn't translate well to boxing).

- Overtraining (sparring too much, leading to early burnout).

- Avoiding strength training (believing it makes fighters slow or bulky).

But modern sports science has changed the game. Fighters now train with scientific precision to optimize speed, power, endurance, and recovery.

Example: In the past, fighters like Muhammad Ali relied on natural talent and hard work. Today, elite fighters use heart rate tracking, strength data, and recovery metrics to train smarter.

The future of boxing belongs to those who use science to maximize performance.

Technology and Data-Driven Training in Boxing

New technology allows fighters to train smarter, prevent injuries, and optimize performance.

1. Wearable Performance Trackers

- Heart rate monitors – Helps fighters track effort levels and avoid over training.

- Punch-tracking devices – Measures speed, power, and punch output in real-time.

- Oxygen sensors – Tracks breathing efficiency to improve endurance.

Example: Fighters like Vasiliy Lomachenko use heart rate monitoring to control their training intensity and recovery.

2. Advanced Recovery & Injury Prevention

The future of boxing isn't just about training harder—it's about recovering better.

- Cryotherapy – Extreme cold therapy reduces muscle inflammation.

- Compression therapy – Improves circulation and speeds up muscle recovery.

- Red light therapy – Helps heal injuries and muscle fatigue faster.

Example: LeBron James and Cristiano Ronaldo spend millions on recovery technology to keep their bodies performing at an elite level. Fighters must adopt the same approach for career longevity.

3. Virtual Reality (VR) & AI Training

Fighters can now train their reaction time, defensive skills, and strategy using technology.

- VR boxing simulations – Allows fighters to simulate real opponents without taking damage.

- AI-assisted training – Customizes workouts based on a fighter's weaknesses.

- Slow-motion punch analysis – Breaks down technique frame-by-frame for improvement.

Example: Future training camps may use VR headsets for advanced reaction training, improving fighters' ability to read opponents.

The New Approach to Strength Training for Fighters

Old-school trainers believed that lifting weights made fighters slow. But today, we know that strength training is essential for:

- More explosive punches

- Better injury resistance

- Increased endurance and durability

The Future of Strength & Conditioning in Boxing

- Olympic-style weightlifting – Power cleans,

snatches, and explosive lifts develop fast-twitch muscle fibers for knockout power.

- Isometric training – Holding resistance in place (e.g., holding a squat position) builds stability and endurance in muscles.

- Velocity-based training (VBT) – Sensors track bar speed during lifts, ensuring optimal force development.

- Reactive strength training – Plyometrics combined with weighted resistance improves speed and movement efficiency.

Example: Fighters like Saul "Canelo" Álvarez incorporate strength training and explosive lifts without sacrificing speed.

Mistake: Fighters who ignore modern strength training techniques will fall behind those who train smarter.

Aerobic vs. Anaerobic Training: The Future of Boxing Cardio

Traditional boxing training relied heavily on roadwork (long-distance running), but sports science has proven that:

- Too much slow running reduces explosive power.

- Boxing requires anaerobic endurance, not marathon stamina.

The New Approach to Cardio for Boxing

- Sprint intervals – 100-400m sprints build fight-specific endurance.

- Explosive footwork drills – Improves agility and stamina at the same time.

- Energy system testing – Determines if a fighter needs more aerobic or anaerobic work.

Example: The best fighters now train short bursts of intense effort, mimicking fight conditions.

Mistake: Fighters who do too much slow running may find themselves gassing out in explosive fights.

Customized Training Plans for Individual Fighters

The future of boxing training is not one-size-fits-all. Fighters are learning that each body type and fighting style needs a customized training plan.

Tailoring Training to a Fighter's Body Type

- Ectomorphs (Lean & Long Fighters) → Need more strength work and explosive power training.

- Mesomorphs (Naturally Athletic Fighters) → Need balance of strength, speed, and endurance training.

- Endomorphs (Stocky, Heavyweight Fighters)
  → Need more speed and agility training to stay mobile.

Example: A heavyweight like Tyson Fury focuses on agility drills, while a lightweight like Gervonta Davis emphasizes explosive power.

Mistake: Fighters who train like everyone else instead of customizing their program won't reach their full potential.

What the Next Generation of Fighters Must Do to Stay Ahead

The best fighters of the future won't just rely on talent—they will train with cutting-edge methods.

The Future Champion's Training Blueprint

- Use data & technology – Track punch speed, heart rate, and reaction time.

- Train smarter, not just harder – Prioritize explosive training over excessive endurance work.

- Recover like an elite athlete – Use nutrition, sleep, and therapy to stay in top shape.

- Adapt to new training methods – Fighters who resist change will get left behind.

Example: Floyd Mayweather's training methods were ahead of his time—future fighters must evolve even further.

Mistake: Fighters who stick to outdated training methods will be outclassed by those who use sports science and technology.

Conclusion: The Future Belongs to Those Who Adapt

Boxing is entering a new era of training, where science, technology, and smart conditioning will create the next generation of champions.

- Those who train with data, technology, and advanced methods will dominate.

- The old-school way is evolving—fighters must adapt or fall behind.

- Strength & conditioning will play an even bigger role in boxing's future.

- The best fighters will be explosive, durable, and scientifically prepared for war.

CHAPTER 12
Becoming a Champion: The Legacy of Strength & Conditioning in Boxing

Throughout this book, we have explored the evolution of strength and conditioning in boxing, from the early days of the sport to the cutting-edge training methods shaping today's champions. But at the heart of it all, one truth remains:

Champions are not born; they are built.

This final chapter will summarize everything it takes to become a champion, from the mental and physical preparation to the daily discipline that separates the great from the average. This is the legacy of strength and conditioning in boxing—and the blueprint for success.

The Formula for a Champion

A champion isn't just someone with skill, power, or speed—they are fighters who have mastered all aspects of training, discipline, and mindset.

The Four Pillars of a True Champion:

1. Unbreakable Mentality

- Confidence – Believing in yourself, even when no one else does.

- Focus – Staying locked in, avoiding distractions.

- Composure – Staying calm under pressure, never panicking.

- Resilience – Getting up after a knockdown, pushing through pain.

Example: Muhammad Ali mentally defeated his opponents before they even stepped into the ring.

Mistake: A fighter who doubts themselves will never reach the top.

2. Elite Strength & Conditioning

- Explosive Power – Strength training to develop knockout punches.

- Speed & Agility – Footwork drills to move efficiently in the ring.

- Endurance – Energy system training to go 12 rounds at full pace.

- Injury Prevention – Mobility work, recovery, and strength training to prolong a career.

Example: Modern fighters like Canelo Álvarez combine

boxing skills with scientific strength training to optimize their performance.

Mistake: Fighters who avoid strength training will be out-muscled and lack explosive power.

3. Smart Training & Recovery

- Intelligent training – Following structured programs based on sports science.

- Proper recovery – Prioritizing sleep, nutrition, and therapy to stay fresh.

- Year-round conditioning – Staying in shape even when not in fight camp.

Example: Floyd Mayweather stayed in shape year-round, ensuring he never had to "get in shape" for a fight—he was always ready.

Mistake: Fighters who overtrain without proper recovery burn out early.

4. Championship Lifestyle & Discipline

- Consistent hard work – Training like a champion every single day.

- Healthy nutrition – Fueling the body for peak performance.

- Avoiding distractions – Staying away from negative influences.

- Continuous learning – Always improving, evolving, and adapting.

Example: Bernard Hopkins fought at a world-class level until age 50 because he lived like a champion every single day.

Mistake: Many fighters get lazy and undisciplined between fights, ruining their careers.

The Legacy of Strength & Conditioning in Boxing

The history of boxing strength and conditioning has evolved from raw, unstructured training to a scientific approach that maximizes performance.

Early Boxing (17th-20th Century) – Fighters relied only on natural talent and basic conditioning.

Mid-20th Century – Strength training was misunderstood, and boxers avoided lifting weights.

Modern Era (1990s-Present) – Sports science revolutionized boxing training, blending strength, speed, endurance, and recovery.

The Future – The next generation of fighters will use technology, data tracking, and advanced recovery methods to optimize performance.

The fighters who embrace modern strength & conditioning will dominate the sport. Those who ignore it will fall behind.

FINAL WORDS
The Champion's Mindset

The road to becoming a champion is not easy. It takes years of discipline, sacrifice, and relentless effort.

But the truth is this:

- The best fighters are the ones who refuse to make excuses.

- They show up every day, put in the work, and never stop improving.

- They take care of their bodies, train smart, and live like champions—24/7.

- If you want to be great, it's not just about training for a fight. It's about training for life.

Champions aren't made in the ring. They are made in the gym, in the kitchen, in their mindset, and in their daily habits.

So, the question is:

Are you willing to do what it takes to be a champion?

The Path to Greatness Starts Now

This book has laid out the blueprint for strength and conditioning in boxing—the history, the science, and the methods that shape the greatest fighters in the world.

- Now it's up to you to apply it.

- Train smart. Recover properly. Stay disciplined.

- And most importantly—never stop improving.

- The next champion isn't just the most talented fighter—it's the one who is the most prepared.

The question is: Will that be you?

Thank you for reading!

Now go train like a Champion!

ABOUT LARRY WADE

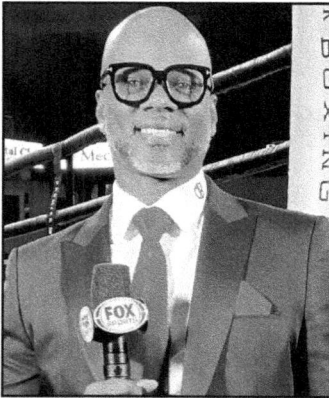

Coach Larry Wade is a world-renowned strength and conditioning coach, former elite track and field athlete, and a celebrated leader in athletic performance development. Wade's journey began in collegiate track and field at Texas A&M University, where he had an undefeated senior season, winning two NCAA National Championships, earning five All-American honors, and securing four Big 12 Conference titles plus a Southwest Conference title. His excellence earned him induction into the Texas A&M Athletic Hall of Fame in 2008.

Following college, Wade received a sponsorship contract from Nike and competed professionally. He rose to rank among the top five hurdlers in the world from 1999 to 2004. His professional highlights include:

- Winning a gold medal at the 2003 Pan American Games,

- Earning a bronze medal at the Goodwill Games,

- And reaching the finals at the World Championships.

After retiring from professional competition, Wade transitioned into coaching.

He first began working with professional track and field athletes, coaching some of the world's best, including:

- Dominique Arnold – American Record Holder in the 110-meter hurdles, World Championship Medalist

- Carmelita Jeter – Olympian, World Champion Sprinter, World Record Holder (4x100-meter relay)

- Candice Davis – World Championship Medalist (60m hurdles)

- Rodney Martin – Olympian (200m, 4x100m relay)

- Shevon Stoddart – Olympian (400m hurdles)

- Uhunoma Osazuwa – Olympian, National Record Holder (heptathlon)

Building on his success in track and field, Wade expanded into performance coaching for NFL athletes, enhancing the speed, strength, and conditioning of several notable players, including:

- Chauncey Washington – NFL Running Back (Jacksonville Jaguars, Dallas Cowboys, St. Louis Rams)

- Brandon Manumaleuna – NFL Tight End (St. Louis Rams, San Diego Chargers, Chicago Bears)

- Brian Price – NFL Defensive Tackle (Tampa Bay Buccaneers, Dallas Cowboys, Cleveland Browns)

- Javorius "Buck" Allen – NFL Running Back (Baltimore Ravens, New Orleans Saints)

- Quinton Pointer – NFL Cornerback (St. Louis Rams, Tampa Bay Buccaneers)

- Devante Davis – NFL Wide Receiver (Philadelphia Eagles)

- Thomas Graham Jr. – NFL Cornerback (Chicago Bears)

Following his success with NFL athletes, Wade transitioned into professional boxing strength and conditioning, where he has become one of the most sought-after coaches in combat sports.

Coach Wade has trained a powerhouse roster of world champions and elite fighters, including:

- Shawn Porter (WBC and IBF Welterweight World Champion)

- Badou Jack (WBC Super Middleweight World Champion, WBA Light Heavyweight World Champion, WBC Cruiserweight World Champion)

- Caleb Plant (IBF Super Middleweight World Champion)

- Luis Ortiz (WBA Interim Heavyweight World Champion)

- Robeisy Ramirez (WBO Featherweight World Champion, Two-time Olympic Gold Medalist)

- Rolando Romero (WBA Interim Lightweight World Champion and WBA Lightweight World Champion)

- Patrick Teixeira (WBO Super Welterweight World Champion)

- Kazuto Ioka (WBO Super Flyweight World Champion, Four-Division World Champion)

- Marlon Tapales (Unified Super Bantamweight World Champion)

- Joe Joyce (WBO Interim Heavyweight World Champion)

- Shane Mosley Sr. (Three-Division World Champion, Former WBC, WBA, and IBF Champion)

He has also coached other top contenders, rising stars, and crossover athletes, including:

- Jake Paul (Professional boxer and global crossover athlete)

- Shane Mosley Jr. (Middleweight contender)

- Olajide "KSI" Olatunji (Crossover entertainer and professional boxer)

- Jesus Ramos Jr. (Super Welterweight contender)

- Blair "The Flair" Cobbs (Welterweight contender)

- Marcela Cornejo (Super Middleweight World Title Challenger)

Wade's scientific approach — blending speed development, strength training, explosive conditioning, and injury prevention — has been widely credited for elevating the careers of his athletes.

His work has been featured in major media outlets such as the *New York Times, Yahoo Sports,* and the *Sun Times,* cementing his influence on athletic performance across multiple sports.

In recognition of his extraordinary contributions, the City of Las Vegas officially proclaimed December 15th as *"Coach Larry Wade Day,"* honoring both his athletic excellence and his positive impact on the local and global communities.

Coach Larry Wade is married to Yvonne Wade, the Athletic Director at the College of Southern Nevada. Together, they have two sons, Jordan and Brandon.

Today, Coach Larry Wade continues to build champions, shape legacies, and inspire the next generation of athletes worldwide.

www.ingramcontent.com/pod-product-compliance
Lightning Source LLC
Chambersburg PA
CBHW060242030426
42335CB00014B/1570